FATTY LIVER DIET COOKBOOK FOR NEWLY DIAGNOSED

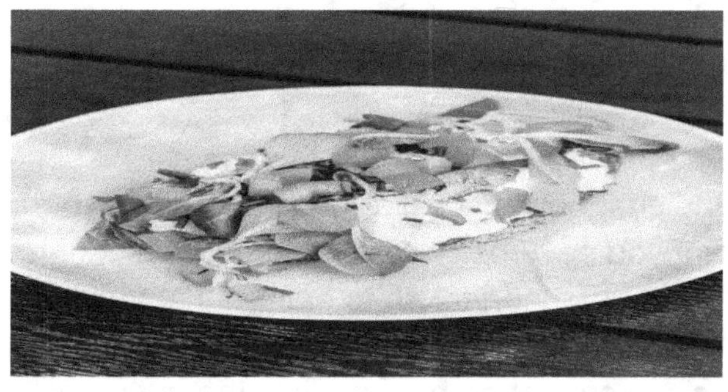

A complete guidelines and recipes to help improve your health and detoxify your liver

Avila Wanda

TABLE OF CONTENTS

Introduction

In the quiet humdrum of everyday life, Avila found herself facing an unexpected twist – a diagnosis that echoed through her world like a distant storm. Fatty liver disease had cast its shadow upon her health, urging her to reevaluate the choices on her plate. As she navigated the maze of medical advice and dietary restrictions, Avila discovered the transformative power of a well-crafted cookbook.

In the midst of uncertainty, she embarked on a journey to create a culinary haven for those grappling with a similar diagnosis. The "Nourishing Harmony Cookbook" emerged as a beacon of hope for the newly diagnosed, offering a curated collection of recipes designed to support liver health. From vibrant salads to hearty mains, each dish was a testament to the idea that nourishing the body could be a flavorful adventure.

The cookbook became Avila's labor of love, weaving together not just ingredients but stories of resilience and renewal. As she delved into the realms of nutrition, she realized that embracing a fatty liver diet didn't mean bidding farewell to taste and pleasure. Instead, it opened the door to a world of culinary exploration, where every recipe was a step towards reclaiming control and savoring life.

Within the pages of the cookbook, Avila poured her heart into demystifying the complexities of dietary adjustments. Nutritional insights and expert tips stood side by side with easy-to-follow recipes, creating a roadmap for the journey towards a healthier, more vibrant life. The "Nourishing Harmony Cookbook" wasn't just a compendium of dishes; it was a companion for those navigating the intricate terrain of dietary change.

As the aroma of wholesome meals filled her kitchen, Avila found solace in the simple act of cooking for wellness. The cookbook, a guide and confidante, beckoned others to join her on this gastronomic odyssey, reminding them that a nourishing diet was not a sacrifice but a celebration of life's abundance.

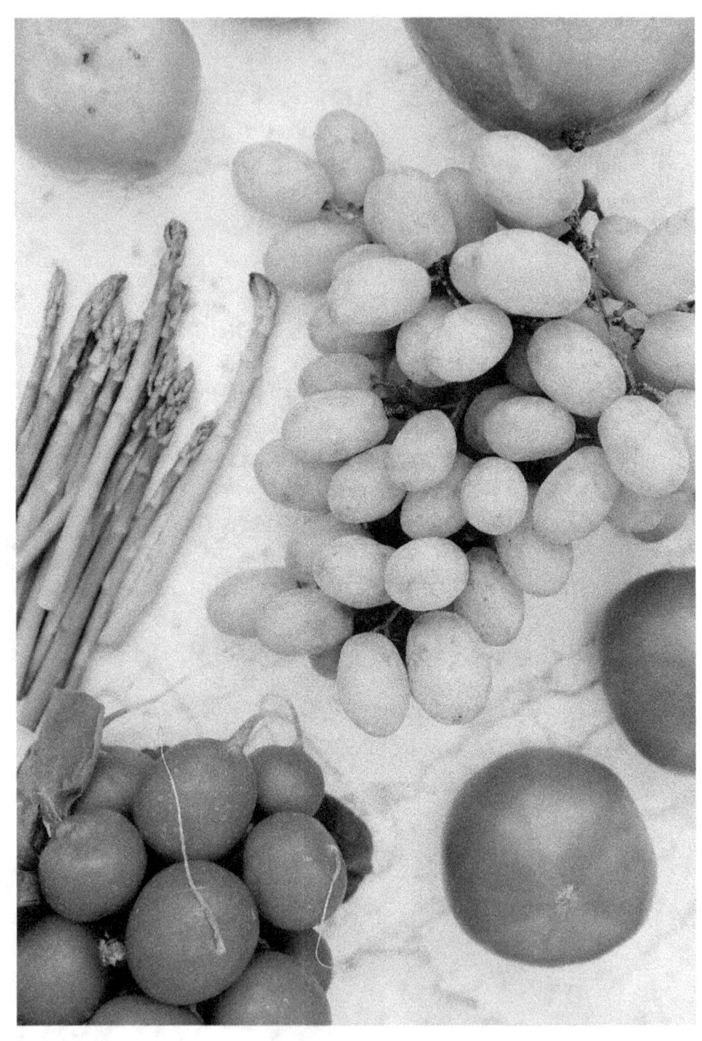

Chapter one

Fatty liver and it's functions

Fatty liver, also known as hepatic steatosis, is a condition characterized by the accumulation of excess fat in liver cells. This can be caused by various factors, including alcohol consumption (alcoholic fatty liver disease) or non-alcoholic factors such as obesity, insulin resistance, high levels of fats in the blood, and certain medications.

Functions of the liver include:

1. Metabolism: The liver plays a crucial role in metabolizing nutrients from the digestive system, including carbohydrates, fats, and proteins. It regulates glucose levels, converts excess glucose into glycogen for

storage, and releases glucose when needed.

2. Detoxification: The liver filters and detoxifies harmful substances, including drugs and toxins, from the blood. It transforms these substances into water-soluble compounds that can be excreted through urine or bile.

3. Synthesis of Proteins: The liver synthesizes various proteins, such as albumin, which helps maintain blood volume and pressure, and clotting factors essential for blood coagulation.

4. Storage of Nutrients: The liver stores essential nutrients, including glycogen, vitamins, and minerals.When the body needs these chemicals, it releases them from storage into the bloodstream.

When the liver undergoes fatty infiltration, it can affect these functions:

1. Impaired Metabolism: Excessive fat in liver cells may interfere with the normal metabolic processes, leading to insulin resistance and dysregulation of glucose and lipid metabolism.

2. Inflammation: Fatty liver can progress to non-alcoholic steatohepatitis (NASH), characterized by inflammation and liver cell damage. This can eventually lead to more severe conditions such as cirrhosis and liver failure.

3. Reduced Detoxification: The accumulation of fat may compromise the liver's ability to efficiently detoxify the blood, potentially allowing harmful substances to build up in the body.

4. Altered Protein Synthesis: Fatty liver can impact the synthesis of proteins, affecting the production of crucial components like albumin and clotting factors.

It's important to address the underlying causes of fatty liver, as prolonged inflammation and damage can lead to serious liver diseases. Lifestyle changes, including a balanced diet, regular exercise, and weight management, are often recommended to manage and prevent fatty liver disease. In cases of alcoholic fatty liver disease, alcohol cessation is crucial for treatment.

Chapter two

Foods to eat and avoids for healthy liver

Foods to Eat for a Healthy Liver:

1. Leafy Greens: Incorporate vegetables like spinach, kale, and broccoli, which are rich in antioxidants and can support liver health.
2. Cruciferous Vegetables: Include broccoli, Brussels sprouts, and cauliflower as they contain compounds that aid in detoxification.
3. Fruits: Opt for fruits such as berries, grapefruit, and apples that are high in antioxidants and fiber, promoting overall liver health.
4. Healthy Fats: Choose sources of healthy fats like avocados, olive oil, and fatty fish (salmon, mackerel) that provide omega-3 fatty acids beneficial for the liver.
5. Nuts and Seeds: Almonds, walnuts, and flaxseeds are rich in omega-3s and antioxidants, supporting liver function.

6. Whole Grains: Include whole grains like brown rice, quinoa, and oats for fiber, which aids in digestion and helps maintain a healthy weight.
7. Lean Proteins: Opt for lean protein sources such as poultry, fish, tofu, and legumes to support liver function without excessive saturated fats.
8. Green Tea: This beverage contains antioxidants that may have protective effects on the liver.
9. Turmeric: Incorporate turmeric into your diet for its anti-inflammatory properties, which can benefit liver health.

Foods to Avoid or Limit:

1. Processed Foods: Reduce intake of processed and packaged foods high in unhealthy fats, sugars, and additives.
2. Fried Foods: Minimize consumption of fried and greasy foods, as they can contribute to weight gain and liver fat accumulation.
3. High-Sugar Foods: Cut down on sugary beverages, sweets, and desserts, as excess sugar can contribute to fatty liver disease.

4. Excessive Salt: Limit salt intake to prevent water retention and potential complications related to liver health.
5. Alcohol: Avoid or limit alcohol consumption, as it can lead to alcoholic liver disease and exacerbate existing liver conditions.
6. Red and Processed Meats: Limit red meat and processed meat intake, as they may contribute to inflammation and liver damage.
7. Artificial Sweeteners: Be cautious with artificial sweeteners, as some studies suggest a potential link to liver issues.
8. High-Caffeine Beverages: While moderate coffee consumption may have potential benefits, excessive caffeine intake should be avoided.

Maintaining a balanced, varied diet, staying hydrated, and adopting a healthy lifestyle are essential for promoting liver health. Individual dietary needs may vary, so it's advisable to consult with a healthcare professional or a registered dietitian for personalized guidance

based on your specific health conditions.

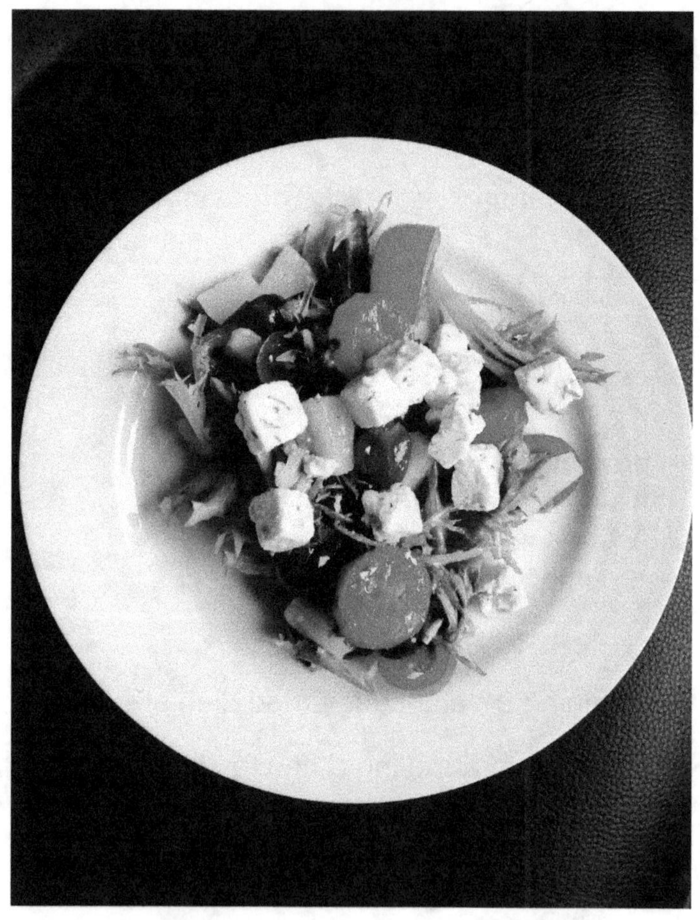

Chapter three

Breakfast Recipes

1. Oatmeal with Berries:

- Cook oats with water or a milk alternative.
- Top with a handful of antioxidant-rich berries like blueberries or raspberries.
- Sprinkle with chia seeds or flaxseeds for added omega-3 fatty acids.

2. Greek Yogurt Parfait:

- Layer Greek yogurt with slices of fresh fruit like kiwi, strawberries, and banana.
- Add a sprinkle of nuts (almonds or walnuts) for healthy fats and crunch.

- For sweetness, drizzle a little honey over the dish.

3. Veggie Omelette:

- Whisk eggs and cook with a variety of colorful vegetables like spinach, bell peppers, and tomatoes.
- Use olive oil for cooking to incorporate healthy fats.
- Serve with avocado slices or whole grain bread.

4. Quinoa Breakfast Bowl:

- Cook quinoa and top with sliced mango, pineapple, and a handful of pomegranate seeds.

- Mix in a dollop of Greek yogurt for creaminess.
- Sprinkle with pumpkin seeds for added nutrients.

5. Avocado Toast with Smoked Salmon:

- Spread mashed avocado on whole grain toast.
- Top with smoked salmon for a dose of omega-3 fatty acids.
- Garnish with a squeeze of lemon juice and fresh herbs like dill.

6. Smoothie Bowl:

- Blend a mixture of spinach, kale, banana, and berries with a base of almond milk.

- Pour into a bowl and add toppings like granola, sliced almonds, and coconut flakes.

7. Chia Seed Pudding:

- Mix chia seeds with almond milk and let it sit in the refrigerator overnight.
- In the morning, layer the pudding with slices of mango, kiwi, and a sprinkle of nuts.

8. Whole Grain Pancakes with Fruit:

- Prepare pancakes using whole grain flour or oats.
- Top with fresh fruit like sliced peaches, strawberries, or apples.

- Use a moderate amount of natural sweeteners like maple syrup.

Remember to focus on whole, nutrient-dense foods, limit added sugars and processed ingredients, and consider incorporating foods that support liver health, such as those rich in antioxidants, fiber, and healthy fats.

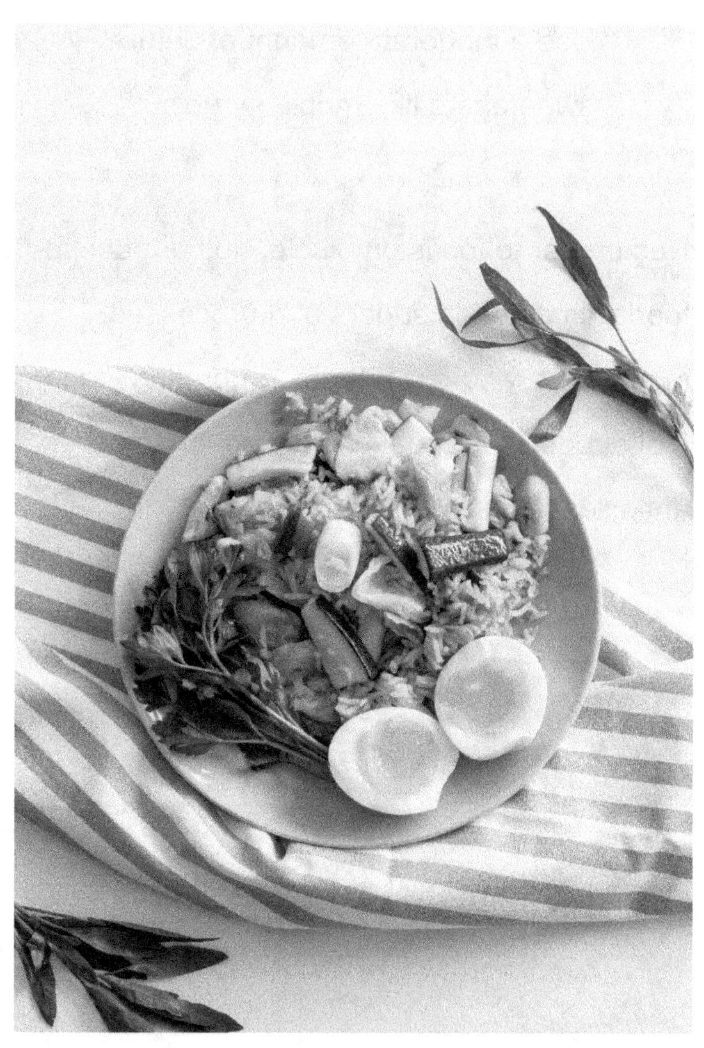

Chapter four

Soups and Stew

Soups and Stews for Fatty Liver Diet:

1. Vegetable Broth:

- Create a hearty vegetable broth using a variety of colorful vegetables like carrots, celery, onions, and leafy greens.
- Add herbs such as thyme and rosemary for flavor without excess salt.
- Use the broth as a base for other soups or stews.

2. Lentil Soup:

- Cook lentils with vegetables like tomatoes, carrots, and spinach.

- Lentils are a good source of protein and
  fiber, promoting satiety and stable blood
  sugar levels.

3. Quinoa and Vegetable Stew:

- Combine quinoa with a mix of
  vegetables such as zucchini, bell
  peppers, and kale.
- Use a low-sodium vegetable broth and
  add herbs like cumin and turmeric for
  added flavor and anti-inflammatory
  benefits.

4. Chicken and Vegetable Soup:

- Prepare a lean chicken soup with plenty
  of vegetables like carrots, celery, and
  broccoli.

- Remove excess fat from the broth to keep it light and heart-healthy.

5. Fish Stew:

- Create a fish stew with a variety of fish such as cod or salmon.
- Add vegetables like tomatoes, onions, and bell peppers for a nutrient-rich meal.

6. Tomato Basil Soup:

- Make a tomato basil soup with fresh tomatoes, garlic, and basil.
- Tomatoes contain antioxidants like lycopene, which may benefit liver health.

7. Spinach and Chickpea Stew:

- Combine chickpeas with spinach, tomatoes, and a mix of spices like cumin and paprika.
- Chickpeas provide plant-based protein and fiber.

8. Miso Soup:

- Prepare miso soup with low-sodium miso paste, tofu, seaweed, and green onions.
- Miso contains probiotics that can support gut health, indirectly benefiting the liver.

Tips for Fatty Liver-Friendly Soups and Stews:

- Limit Sodium: Use low-sodium broths and avoid excessive salt. Herbs and spices can enhance flavor without adding sodium.
- Choose Lean Proteins: Opt for lean protein sources such as chicken, fish, or plant-based proteins like lentils and chickpeas.
- Incorporate Healthy Fats: Add a touch of olive oil or avocado for healthy fats.
- Include Fiber-Rich Ingredients: Vegetables, legumes, and whole grains contribute fiber, promoting digestive health.

- Avoid Creamy Soups: Cream-based
  soups can be high in saturated fats. Opt
  for broth-based or pureed vegetable
  soups.

Maintaining a well-balanced and nutritious diet
is crucial for managing fatty liver disease.
Incorporating these soups and stews into your
meal plan can provide essential nutrients while
supporting liver health.

Chapter five

Salads

Salads for Fatty Liver Diet:

1. Green Leafy Salad with Citrus Vinaigrette:

- Combine mixed greens like spinach, kale, and arugula.
- Add segments of citrus fruits such as oranges or grapefruits.
- Drizzle with a vinaigrette made with olive oil, lemon juice, and a touch of honey.

2. Avocado and Tomato Salad:

- Dice ripe tomatoes and avocados.

- Toss with fresh basil leaves and a sprinkle of pumpkin seeds.
- Dress with a light balsamic vinaigrette.

3. Quinoa and Vegetable Salad:

- Mix cooked quinoa with colorful vegetables like bell peppers, cucumbers, and cherry tomatoes.
- Add fresh herbs like parsley and mint.
- Dress with a lemon-tahini dressing for a burst of flavor.

4. Beet and Walnut Salad:

- Roast or boil beets and slice them into thin rounds.
- Combine with mixed greens, crumbled feta cheese, and chopped walnuts.

- Drizzle with a balsamic glaze.

- Steam broccoli florets and mix with chickpeas.
- Add cherry tomatoes, red onion, and a light yogurt-based dressing.
- Sprinkle with sunflower seeds for added crunch.

- Shred red and green cabbage and toss with sliced apples.
- Add a small handful of dried cranberries or raisins.
- Dress with a yogurt or mustard-based dressing.

7. Spinach and Strawberry Salad:

- Combine fresh spinach with sliced strawberries and cucumber.
- Top with crumbled goat cheese and almonds.
- Drizzle with a poppyseed dressing.

8. Mediterranean Chickpea Salad:

- Mix chickpeas with cherry tomatoes, cucumber, red onion, and Kalamata olives.
- Toss with feta cheese and a lemon-olive oil dressing.
- Sprinkle with oregano for a Mediterranean flair.

Tips for Fatty Liver-Friendly Salads:

- Include Lean Proteins: Add grilled chicken, turkey, or tofu to increase protein content.

- Use Healthy Fats: Incorporate sources of healthy fats such as avocados, nuts, and olive oil.

- Limit Added Sugars: Choose natural sweetness from fruits rather than added sugars in dressings or toppings.

- Experiment with Herbs and Spices: Enhance flavor without adding excessive salt by using herbs like cilantro, mint, or basil.

- Portion Control: Be mindful of portion sizes, and balance your salad with a variety of colorful vegetables.

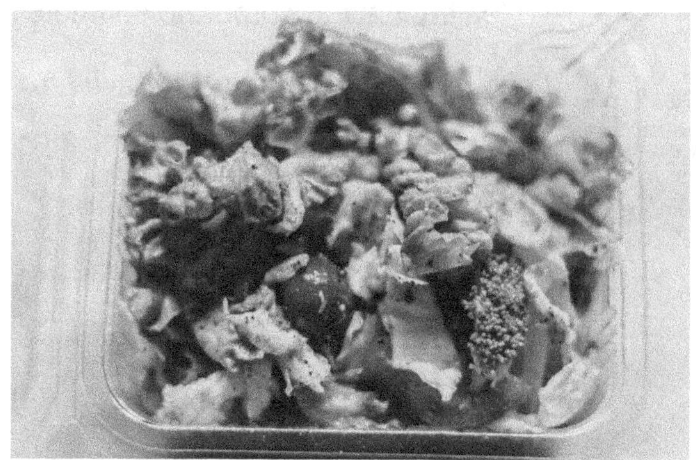

Chapter six

Juices and Smoothies for Fatty Liver Diet:

1. Green Detox Juice:

- Blend kale, spinach, cucumber, celery, and a green apple.
- Squeeze in some lemon juice for a cool variation.
- Consider incorporating a small piece of ginger for its anti-inflammatory properties.

2. Berry Blast Smoothie:

- Blend a mix of berries such as blueberries, strawberries, and raspberries.

- Add Greek yogurt or a plant-based alternative for creaminess.
- Include a handful of spinach for added nutrients.

3. Citrus Sunshine Juice:

- Juice a combination of oranges, grapefruits, and a hint of lime.
- Add a touch of turmeric for its potential anti-inflammatory benefits.
- Dilute with water or coconut water for a lighter option.

4. Tropical Paradise Smoothie:

- Blend pineapple, mango, and kiwi with coconut water.

- Include a tablespoon of chia seeds for omega-3 fatty acids and fiber.
- Optionally, add a splash of aloe vera juice for digestive support.

5. Beet and Carrot Cleanser Juice:

- Juice beets, carrots, and apples for a vibrant, nutrient-rich drink.
- Consider a hint of mint for freshness.
- Dilute with water if the flavors are too intense.

6. Avocado Green Smoothie:

- Blend the avocado, banana, spinach, and almond milk together.
- For an additional protein boost, add a scoop of protein powder.

- Add a touch of honey for sweetness.

7. Cucumber Mint Cooler Juice:

- Juice cucumber and mint leaves for a hydrating and soothing drink.
- Pour in a little lime or lemon juice.
- Serve over ice for a refreshing experience.

8. Anti-Inflammatory Turmeric Smoothie:

- Blend banana, mango, turmeric, and a pinch of black pepper.
- Add coconut milk or almond milk for creaminess.
- Consider adding a tablespoon of flaxseeds for additional omega-3s.

Tips for Fatty Liver-Friendly Juices and Smoothies:

- Limit Added Sugars: Choose naturally sweet fruits to avoid excessive sugar intake.

- Incorporate Fiber: Add ingredients like chia seeds, flaxseeds, or leafy greens for fiber content.

- Hydration is Key: Use water, coconut water, or herbal teas as a base to stay hydrated.

- Mindful Portions: Be mindful of portion sizes, as even healthy juices and smoothies can contribute to calorie intake.

- Experiment with Herbs: Fresh herbs like mint, basil, or cilantro can add flavor without added salt.

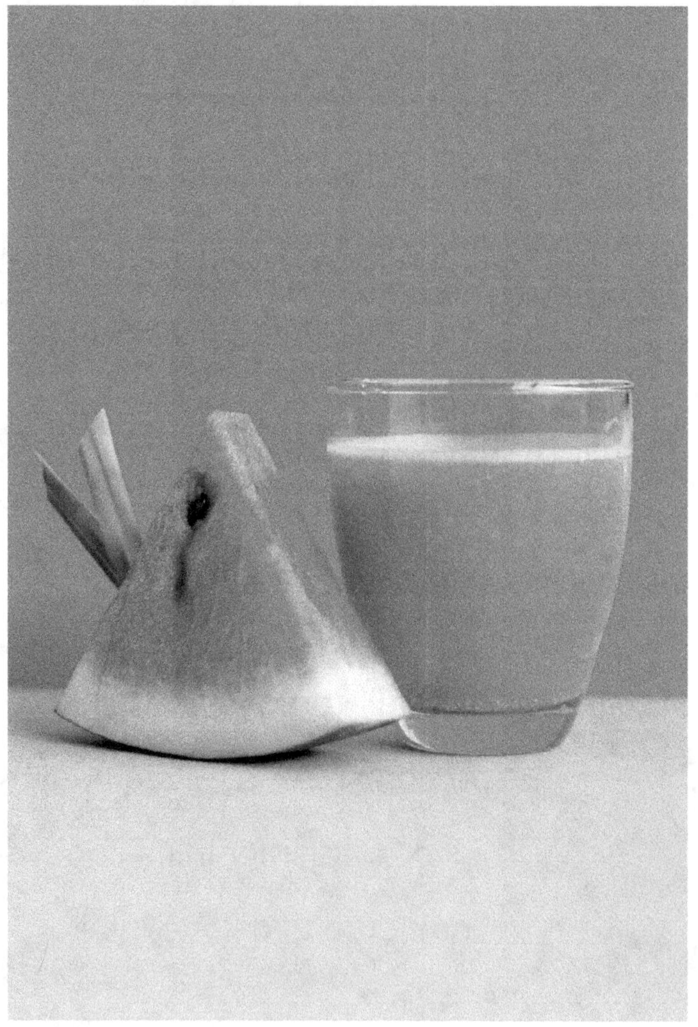

Chapter seven

Desserts

Fruity Chia Seed Pudding:

- Mix chia seeds with unsweetened almond milk and let it thicken in the refrigerator.
- Add a layer of mixed berries (blueberries, raspberries, and strawberries).
- Top with a dollop of Greek yogurt for creaminess.

Baked Apples with Cinnamon:

- Core and slice apples, then toss with a sprinkle of cinnamon.
- Bake until tender.

- Serve with a drizzle of honey and a
  handful of chopped walnuts.

Dark Chocolate-Dipped Strawberries:

- Melt dark chocolate (70% cocoa or
  higher).
- Dip fresh strawberries into the melted
  chocolate.
- Before eating, let them harden and cool.

Yogurt Parfait with Nuts and Berries:

- Layer Greek yogurt with a mix of berries
  (blueberries, raspberries).
- Add a sprinkle of chopped almonds or
  walnuts for crunch.
- For sweetness, drizzle a little honey
  over the dish.

Chia Seed and Mango Sorbet:

- Blend frozen mango chunks with coconut water until smooth.
- Mix in chia seeds and let it set in the freezer until it reaches a sorbet consistency.

Baked Pears with Ricotta:

- Halve and core pears, then bake until tender.
- Fill the center with a spoonful of ricotta cheese.
- Sprinkle some cinnamon on top and drizzle with some honey.

Mixed Berry Smoothie Bowl:

- Blend a mix of berries with a banana and almond milk.
- Pour into a bowl and top with granola, shredded coconut, and a few fresh berries.

Cinnamon and Walnut Oat Bars:

- Combine rolled oats, chopped walnuts, and a dash of cinnamon.
- Mix with mashed bananas and bake into bars.
- Cut into squares and enjoy as a wholesome dessert.

Tips for Fatty Liver-Friendly Desserts:

- Choose Natural Sweeteners: Opt for natural sweeteners like honey, maple syrup, or the natural sweetness of fruits.

- Portion Control: Enjoy desserts in moderation to manage calorie intake.

- Incorporate Healthy Fats: Use nuts, seeds, or avocados for added richness and nutritional benefits.

- Mindful Baking: When baking,
  consider using whole grain flour or
  alternative flours for a healthier
  option.

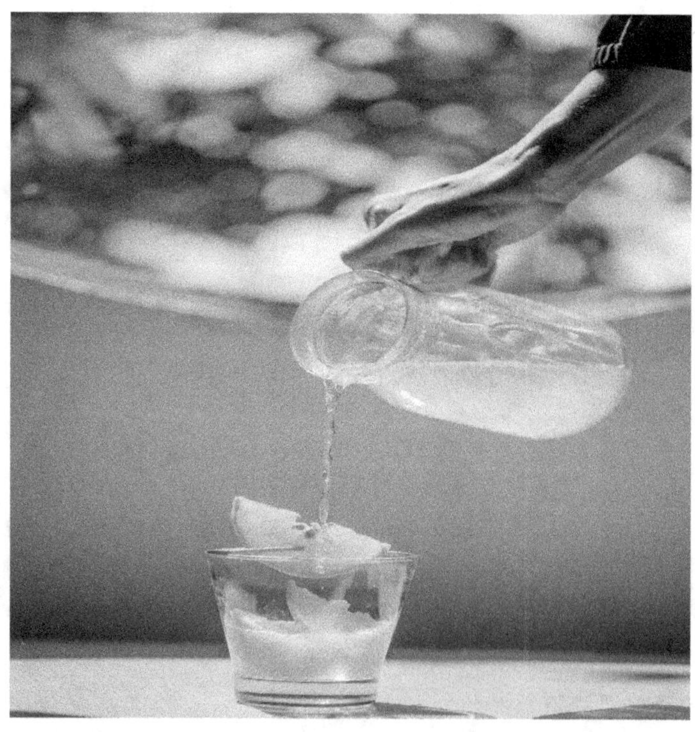

Chapter eight

Grains and legumes

Grains for Fatty Liver Diet:

1. Quinoa:
   - Rich in protein and fiber, quinoa is a versatile grain that can be used as a base for salads, bowls, or a side dish.

2. Brown Rice:
   - A whole grain option with fiber and essential nutrients, brown rice can be a healthier alternative to white rice.

3. Oats:
   - High in soluble fiber, oats can help lower cholesterol levels.

They are great for breakfast as oatmeal or added to smoothies.

4. Barley:

    o   Contains beta-glucans, a type of soluble fiber that may support heart health. Barley can be served as a side dish or added to soups and stews.

5. Buckwheat:

    o   Despite its name, buckwheat is gluten-free and provides a good source of protein and fiber. It can be used in porridge or as a substitute for traditional grains.

6. Millet:

    o   A gluten-free grain with a mildly sweet flavor. Millet can be used in salads, as a side dish, or in place of rice in certain recipes.

7. Whole Wheat:

   o Choose whole wheat products
     like whole wheat bread, pasta, or
     couscous for added fiber and
     nutrients.

8. Farro:

   o An ancient grain with a nutty
     flavor, farro is rich in fiber,
     protein, and nutrients. It works
     well as a side dish or in salads
     and soups.

Legumes for Fatty Liver Diet:

1. Lentils:

   o Packed with protein and fiber,
     lentils are versatile and can be
     used in soups, stews, salads, or
     as a meat substitute.

2. Chickpeas:

    o   A good source of plant-based
        protein and fiber, chickpeas can
        be roasted for snacks, added to
        salads, or used to make
        hummus.

3. Black Beans:

    o   High in fiber and protein, black
        beans are suitable for salads,
        wraps, or as a side dish. They
        can also be blended into soups or
        dips.

4. Kidney Beans:

    o   Rich in antioxidants and fiber,
        kidney beans are commonly used
        in chili, salads, or as a side dish.

5. Edamame:

    o   Young soybeans are a good
        source of protein and can be

enjoyed as a snack, added to

salads, or included in stir-fries.

6. Split Peas:

   ○ High in fiber and protein, split

   peas are commonly used in

   soups and stews.

7. Cannellini Beans:

   ○ These white beans are a good

   source of protein and can be

   used in salads, soups, or as a

   side dish.

8. Green Peas:

   ○ Rich in fiber, green peas can be

   added to salads, rice dishes, or

   enjoyed as a side.

Tips for Fatty Liver-Friendly Grains and Legumes:

- Choose Whole Grains: Opt for whole grains over refined grains for increased fiber and nutrient content.
- Regulate Portion Sizes: To control calorie consumption, pay attention to portion sizes.
- Experiment with Herbs and Spices: Enhance flavor without added salt by using herbs and spices.
- Limit Added Fats: When cooking grains and legumes, use healthy cooking methods and limit added fats.
- Stay Hydrated: Adequate water intake is essential, especially when consuming a high-fiber diet.

Conclusion

In concluding this Fatty Liver Diet Cookbook for the newly diagnosed, remember that the journey toward a healthier liver is not just a series of dietary changes but a commitment to nurturing your overall well-being. Embrace the abundance of wholesome foods that support liver health, from vibrant fruits and vegetables to nutrient-packed grains and legumes. As you explore the delightful recipes within these pages, savor the knowledge that each bite is a step toward rejuvenating your body.

This cookbook is not just a collection of recipes; it's a guide to a lifestyle that embraces balance, moderation, and the joy of nourishing yourself with foods that promote healing. Harness the power of whole foods, mindful cooking, and the personalized approach to find what truly works for you. Recall that progress, not perfection, is the goal of this trip.

As you embark on this path, consult with healthcare professionals, listen to your body, and celebrate the small victories along the way. Your commitment to a fatty liver-friendly diet is an investment in your health, and with each mindful choice, you pave the way for a brighter, healthier future.

May these recipes not only tantalize your taste buds but also serve as a compass guiding you toward optimal liver health and a life filled with vitality. Here's to a journey of wellness, resilience, and a thriving, nourished you.